Stress Management

STRESS MANAGEMENT

The Escape Route From a Silent Killer

Stress Management

George G. Porter

COPYRIGHT PAGE

brief quotations embodied in critical reviews and certain other noncommercial uses permitted by copyright law.

TABLE OF CONTENT

INTRODUCTION

In the fast-paced whirlwind of modern life, stress has become an all-too-familiar companion. It lurks in the shadows, silently infiltrating our minds and bodies and wreaking havoc on our well-being. Yet, despite its pervasive presence, stress often goes unnoticed until its effects manifest in physical or mental health ailments. This silent killer knows no boundaries, affecting individuals of all ages, backgrounds, and walks of life. However, there is hope—a beacon of light in the darkness. Stress management offers an escape route, a pathway to reclaiming control over our lives and restoring harmony to our minds and bodies. In this exploration of stress management, we delve into the depths of this silent killer, uncovering strategies and techniques to navigate its treacherous waters and emerge stronger, healthier, and more resilient than ever before. Join us on this journey as we embark on the quest for inner peace and well-being in a world besieged by stress.

CHAPTER 1: Understanding Stress

Stress is the body's natural response to perceived threats or challenges. It triggers a cascade of physiological and psychological reactions aimed at preparing us to deal with the perceived danger, commonly known as the fight-or-flight response. While stress can be a normal part of life and can even be beneficial in small doses, chronic or excessive stress can have detrimental effects on our physical and mental health.

Types of stress:

1. Acute stress: This type of stress is short-term and often arises from specific situations or events, such as an upcoming exam, a job interview, or a deadline at work. Acute stress typically dissipates once the stressor is removed or the situation is resolved.

2. Chronic Stress: Chronic stress results from prolonged exposure to stressors, such as ongoing financial problems, relationship issues, or work-related pressure. Unlike acute stress, chronic stress persists over an extended period and can have serious implications for health if left unmanaged.

3. Episodic Acute Stress:Some individuals experience acute stress on a frequent basis, often due to their personality traits, lifestyle, or circumstances. This pattern of episodic acute

stress can lead to a cycle of recurring stressors and may increase the risk of developing chronic health problems if not addressed.

4. Traumatic Stress:Traumatic stress occurs in response to traumatic events such as natural disasters, accidents, or violence. It can have profound and long-lasting effects on a person's mental and emotional well-being, often requiring specialized intervention and support.

Causes of stress:

1. External Stressors:These are factors in the external environment that trigger stress reactions. Common external stressors include work pressures, financial difficulties, relationship problems, major life changes (such as moving or starting a new job), and exposure to traumatic events.

2. Internal Stressors: Internal stressors originate from within the individual and often involve self-imposed pressure, unrealistic expectations, perfectionism, or negative thought patterns. Internal stressors can be just as impactful as external ones and may contribute to chronic stress if not addressed.

3. Physiological Stressors:Certain physiological factors, such as illness, injury, lack of sleep, poor nutrition, or hormonal imbalances, can contribute to stress. These internal disruptions can exacerbate the body's stress response and make it more difficult to cope with external stressors.

4. Psychological Stressors:Psychological stressors stem from cognitive or emotional sources, such as worry, fear, anxiety, depression, or unresolved trauma. These internal struggles can intensify the stress experience and may require psychological interventions to address underlying issues.

Understanding the various types and causes of stress is the first step toward effective stress management. By recognizing the sources of stress in our lives, we can begin to implement strategies to mitigate its impact and promote greater resilience and well-being.

CHAPTER 2: The Impact of Stress on Health

Stress is a natural response to challenging situations, but when it becomes chronic, it can wreak havoc on both physical and mental well-being. Understanding its multifaceted impact is crucial for managing and mitigating its effects.

Physical Health

Chronic stress takes a toll on the body, leading to various physical health issues:

1. Cardiovascular Problems: Prolonged stress can elevate blood pressure, increase heart rate, and contribute to the development of heart disease.

2. Immune System Suppression: Stress hormones can suppress the immune system, making

individuals more susceptible to infections and illnesses.

3. Digestive Disorders: Stress can disrupt digestion, leading to issues like irritable bowel syndrome, acid reflux, and stomach ulcers.

4. Musculoskeletal Pain: Tense muscles and poor posture due to stress can result in chronic headaches, back pain, and muscle tension.

Mental Health

The impact of stress on mental health is profound, affecting cognition, mood, and behavior.

1. Anxiety and Depression: Chronic stress is a significant risk factor for anxiety disorders and depression, leading to persistent feelings of worry, sadness, and hopelessness.

2. Cognitive Decline: Prolonged stress can impair memory, concentration, and decision-making abilities, contributing to cognitive decline over time.

3. Sleep Disturbances: Stress often disrupts sleep patterns, resulting in insomnia or poor-quality sleep, which further exacerbates mental health issues.

4. Substance Abuse: Some individuals turn to alcohol, drugs, or other harmful behaviors as coping mechanisms for stress, leading to substance abuse disorders.

Emotional Well-being: Emotional well-being encompasses how individuals perceive, express, and manage their emotions

Mood Swings: Chronic stress can

cause rapid shifts in mood, leading

to irritability, agitation, and

emotional instability

2. Social Withdrawal: Stress may lead individuals to isolate themselves from others, impacting their social relationships and support networks.

3. Low Self-Esteem: Persistent stress can erode self-confidence and self-worth, fostering feelings of inadequacy and self-doubt.

4. Difficulty Coping: High levels of stress can overwhelm coping mechanisms, making it challenging to effectively manage everyday challenges and stressors.

The impact of stress on health is undeniable, affecting every aspect of well-being. Recognizing the signs of stress and implementing healthy coping strategies, such as exercise, relaxation techniques, and seeking social support, are crucial steps in mitigating its negative effects and promoting overall health and resilience.

CHAPTER 3:Recognizing Signs and Symptoms of Stress

Stress can manifest in various ways, impacting both the body and mind. Recognizing the signs and symptoms is the first step in effectively managing stress.

Physical Symptoms

1. Headaches: persistent tension Headaches or migraines can be a physical manifestation of stress.

2. Muscle Tension: Tightness or soreness in the muscles, particularly in the neck, shoulders, and back, can result from stress-induced tension.

3. Fatigue: Feeling constantly tired or lacking energy, despite adequate rest, is a common physical symptom of stress.

4. Gastrointestinal Issues: Stress can lead to digestive problems such as stomach pain, nausea, diarrhea, or constipation.

5. Insomnia: Difficulty falling asleep, staying asleep, or experiencing restful sleep can be indicative of stress-related sleep disturbances.

Emotional Symptoms

1. Anxiety: Persistent feelings of worry, nervousness, or apprehension, even in the absence of a specific threat, may indicate underlying stress.

2. Depression: Intense feelings of sadness, hopelessness, or despair that interfere with daily functioning can be a sign of chronic stress.

3. Irritability: Easily becoming agitated, short-tempered, or having a low tolerance for frustration can be an emotional response to stress.

4. Mood Swings: Rapid and unpredictable shifts in mood, from euphoria to despair, may occur in response to stressors.

5. Difficulty Concentrating: Struggling to focus, remember details, or make decisions can be a cognitive manifestation of stress.

Behavioral Symptoms

1. Changes in Eating Habits: Stress can lead to overeating or loss of appetite, resulting in weight gain or loss.

2. Social withdrawal: Avoiding social interactions, isolating oneself from friends and family, or becoming increasingly reclusive can be behavioral signs of stress.

3. Procrastination: Putting off tasks or responsibilities, even when they are important or time-sensitive, may indicate avoidance behavior driven by stress.

4. Increased Substance Use: Turning to alcohol, drugs, or other substances as a coping mechanism for stress is a maladaptive behavioral response.

5. Restlessness: Feeling restless, fidgety, or unable to relax, even during downtime, can be a behavioral manifestation of underlying stress.

Recognizing the signs and symptoms of stress is crucial for implementing appropriate coping strategies and seeking support when needed. By addressing stress early on and adopting healthy coping mechanisms, individuals can better manage its impact on their physical, emotional, and behavioral well-being

CHAPTER 4:Strategies For Managing Stress

Stress is an inevitable part of life, but how we respond to it can make a significant difference in our overall well-being. Implementing healthy coping strategies can help mitigate the negative effects of stress and promote resilience.

1. Mindfulness and meditation

Practicing mindfulness and meditation can help reduce stress by bringing awareness to the present moment and promoting relaxation. Even just a few minutes of deep breathing or guided meditation each day can have a profound impact on stress levels.

2. Regular Exercise

Engaging in regular physical activity, whether it's walking, jogging, yoga, or dancing, can help reduce stress hormones and release endorphins, the body's natural mood elevators. Aim for at least 30 minutes of exercise most days of the week.

3. Healthy lifestyle habits

Maintaining a healthy lifestyle can support stress management. This includes eating a balanced diet, getting adequate sleep, and avoiding excessive caffeine, alcohol, and nicotine, which can exacerbate stress.

4. Social Support

Seeking support from friends, family, or support groups can provide a sense of connection and belonging, helping to buffer the effects of stress. Talking to someone you trust about your feelings can offer perspective and emotional relief.

5. Time Management

Effective time management can help reduce stress by prioritizing tasks, setting realistic goals, and breaking large tasks into smaller, manageable steps. Learn to delegate tasks when possible and say no to additional commitments when feeling overwhelmed.

6. Relaxation Techniques

Incorporate relaxation techniques such as deep breathing exercises, progressive muscle relaxation, or visualization into your daily routine. These techniques can help calm the mind and body, reducing the physiological symptoms of stress.

7. Set Boundaries

Establishing clear boundaries in both personal and professional relationships is essential for managing stress. Learn to assertively communicate your needs and limits, and don't be afraid to say no to requests that may lead to excessive stress.

8. Seek professional help.

If stress becomes overwhelming or persists despite self-care efforts, don't hesitate to seek professional help from a therapist or counselor. They can provide personalized strategies and support to help you better manage stress and improve your overall well-being.

By incorporating these strategies into your daily life, you can effectively manage stress and cultivate resilience in the face of life's challenges. Remember that it's okay to ask for help when needed and to prioritize self-care to maintain your physical, emotional, and mental health.

Chapter 4.1: Timely and adequate sex in optimal stress management

The Role of Timely and Adequate Sex in Optimal Stress Management

Sexual activity is not only a pleasurable aspect of human relationships but also plays a significant role in promoting overall well-being, including stress management. Understanding how sex can contribute to stress relief and implementing healthy sexual practices can enhance both physical and mental health.

1. Stress-Reducing Hormones

During sexual activity, the body releases hormones such as oxytocin, dopamine, and endorphins, often referred to as "feel-good" hormones. These hormones promote feelings of relaxation, pleasure, and happiness, counteracting the effects of stress hormones like cortisol.

2. Physical Relaxation

Engaging in sexual activity, whether alone or with a partner, can lead to physical relaxation by reducing muscle tension and promoting better circulation. This physical release of tension can alleviate the physical symptoms of stress, such as headaches, muscle aches, and fatigue.

3. Improved Mood

Sexual activity has been linked to improved mood and emotional well-being. The intimacy and connection shared during sex can foster feelings of closeness, intimacy, and emotional bonding with a partner, reducing feelings of loneliness and anxiety.

4. Better sleep quality

Sexual activity has been shown to promote better sleep quality, which is essential for overall stress management. The release of hormones like oxytocin and prolactin during orgasm can induce feelings of relaxation and drowsiness, making it easier to fall asleep and stay asleep throughout the night.

5.   Enhanced Relationship Satisfaction

For individuals in committed relationships, regular sexual activity can enhance relationship satisfaction and resilience to stress. The emotional intimacy and communication fostered through sex can strengthen the bond between partners and provide a source of support during challenging times.

6.   Stress Relief Through Self-Exploration

Solo sexual activity, also known as masturbation, can also provide stress relief and promote self-exploration and self-acceptance. Masturbation allows individuals to explore their own bodies, desires, and boundaries, which can lead to increased self-confidence and self-awareness.

7. Communication and Connection

Open communication about sexual desires, preferences, and boundaries with a partner can deepen emotional intimacy and foster a sense of connection. Discussing sexual needs and fantasies in a safe and respectful environment can enhance trust and understanding, reducing relationship-related stress.

8. Consent and respect

It's important to emphasize that sexual activity should always be consensual and respectful. Prioritizing mutual consent, communication, and respect for boundaries is essential for promoting positive sexual experiences and maintaining healthy relationships.

Stress Management

Incorporating timely and adequate sexual activity into your life can be a valuable component of stress management and overall well-being. Whether alone or with a partner, embracing sexuality in a healthy and respectful manner can contribute to physical relaxation, emotional intimacy, and enhanced relationship satisfaction.

CHAPTER 5:Creating Your Personalized Stress Management Plan

Stress is an inevitable part of life, but how we respond to it can greatly influence our well-being. By developing a personalized stress management plan, you can identify effective strategies to cope with stress and promote overall resilience. Here's how to get started:

1. Assess your stressors.

Begin by identifying the sources of stress in your life. These may include work-related pressures, relationship conflicts, financial concerns, health issues, or major life changes. Take stock of both external stressors (such as deadlines or obligations) and internal stressors (such as perfectionism or negative self-talk).

2. Recognize your stress responses.

Next, become aware of how stress manifests in your body, mind, and behavior. Pay attention to physical symptoms (such as headaches or muscle tension), emotional responses (such as anxiety or irritability), and behavioral patterns (such as procrastination or social withdrawal). Understanding your unique stress responses will guide your selection of coping strategies.

3. Identify coping strategies.

Explore a variety of stress management techniques and identify those that resonate with you. These may include:

Mindfulness and Meditation: Practice mindfulness techniques, such as deep breathing exercises or guided meditation, to cultivate present-moment awareness and promote relaxation.

Physical Activity: Engage in regular exercise, whether it's walking, yoga, swimming, or dancing, to reduce stress hormones and boost mood-enhancing endorphins.

Healthy Lifestyle Habits: Prioritize self-care activities such as getting adequate sleep, maintaining a balanced diet, and limiting caffeine and alcohol intake.

Social Support: Seek support from friends, family, or support groups to share your feelings, gain perspective, and receive encouragement during challenging times.

Time Management: Organize your time effectively by setting realistic goals, prioritizing tasks, and breaking larger projects into smaller, manageable steps.

Relaxation Techniques: Incorporate relaxation practices such as progressive muscle relaxation, visualization, or aromatherapy into your daily routine to reduce tension and promote calmness.

Seeking Professional Help: Don't hesitate to consult a therapist, counselor, or healthcare professional if stress becomes overwhelming or interferes with your daily functioning.

4. Create your stress management toolkit.

Compile a list of your chosen coping strategies and techniques into a personalized stress management toolkit. Keep this toolkit easily accessible, whether it's a physical journal, digital document, or mobile app, so you can refer to it whenever you need support.

5. Implement your plan consistently.

Commit to incorporating your chosen stress management techniques into your daily routine. Schedule regular self-care activities, prioritize relaxation, and practice coping strategies proactively, not just when stress becomes overwhelming.

6. Evaluate and adjust.

Periodically evaluate the effectiveness of your stress management plan and adjust as needed. Notice which strategies work best for you and which may need tweaking. Be flexible and willing to experiment with new techniques to find what works best for your unique needs.

By creating a personalized stress management plan tailored to your individual stressors, responses, and preferences, you can build resilience and navigate life's challenges with greater ease. Remember that managing stress is an ongoing process, and prioritizing self-care is key to maintaining overall health and well-being.

5.1:Crafting Your Personalized Stress Management Plan

Creating a personalized stress management plan involves identifying specific stressors in your life and developing strategies to effectively cope with them. Here are the key steps to help you craft your personalized stress management plan:

1. Identify your stressors:

Start by identifying the specific situations, events, or circumstances that trigger stress in your life. These stressors can be related to work, relationships, finances, health, or any other aspect of your life. Take some time to reflect on what causes you stress and write it down.

2. Assess your coping strategies:

Next, assess the coping strategies you currently use to manage stress. Reflect on whether these strategies are effective in reducing your stress levels or if they contribute to more stress in the long run. Consider both healthy coping mechanisms, such as exercise or mindfulness, and unhealthy ones, such as excessive drinking or avoidance.

3. Set realistic goals:

Based on your identified stressors and coping strategies, set realistic goals for managing stress. These goals should be specific, measurable, achievable, relevant, and time-bound (SMART). For example, if one of your stressors is work-related, a goal could be to practice relaxation techniques for 10 minutes every day during your lunch break.

4. Explore stress management techniques:

Explore various stress management techniques and strategies to incorporate into your personalized plan.

This may include relaxation techniques like deep breathing, meditation, progressive muscle relaxation, or activities that promote mindfulness, such as yoga or tai chi. Experiment with different techniques to find what works best for you.

5. Develop healthy habits.

Incorporate healthy habits into your daily routine to support stress management. This includes prioritizing regular physical activity, eating a balanced diet, getting enough sleep, and avoiding excessive alcohol, caffeine, and nicotine. A healthy lifestyle can enhance your resilience to stress and improve your overall well-being.

6. Establish Boundaries:

Set clear boundaries in your personal and professional life to protect your time, energy, and well-being. Learn to say no to activities or commitments that add unnecessary stress to your life, and communicate your boundaries assertively to others.

7. Seek Support:

Don't hesitate to seek support from friends, family members, or a mental health professional if you're struggling to manage stress on your own. Talking to someone you trust can provide emotional support, perspective, and practical advice for coping with stress.

8. Review and Adjust:

Regularly review your stress management plan and assess its effectiveness in reducing your stress levels and improving your overall well-being. Be open to adjusting your plan as needed based on changes in your circumstances or feedback from your experiences.

By following these steps and crafting a personalized stress management plan that addresses your unique needs and preferences, you can develop effective strategies for coping with stress and leading a more balanced and fulfilling life. Remember that managing stress is an ongoing process, and it's essential to prioritize self-care and make adjustments as needed to support your well-being.

5.2:Understanding Stress Triggers:

Stress is an inevitable part of life, but understanding its triggers can empower individuals to manage it effectively. Assessing stress triggers involves a deliberate examination of various factors that contribute to feelings of stress and anxiety. By identifying these triggers, individuals can develop personalized strategies to mitigate their impact and promote emotional well-being.

Identifying Situational Triggers:

Situational triggers are external events or circumstances that induce stress reactions. These can include work deadlines, financial difficulties, conflicts in relationships, or major life changes such as moving or starting a new job. Assessing situational triggers involves recognizing recurring patterns and pinpointing specific situations that consistently lead to stress.

Exploring Emotional Triggers:

Emotional triggers are internal responses to external stimuli that evoke strong emotional reactions. These can include feelings of inadequacy, fear of failure, perfectionism, or unresolved trauma. Assessing emotional triggers involves introspection and self-awareness to recognize the thoughts and emotions that precede stress reactions.

Recognizing behavioral triggers:

Behavioral triggers are habitual responses or coping mechanisms that exacerbate stress. These can include procrastination, overeating, substance abuse, or avoiding social interactions. Assessing behavioral triggers involves observing patterns of behavior and identifying maladaptive coping strategies that contribute to stress.

Utilizing Journaling and Reflection:

Journaling is a powerful tool for assessing stress triggers. By recording daily experiences, thoughts, and emotions, individuals can identify recurring patterns and triggers. Reflecting on journal entries can provide valuable insights into the underlying causes of stress and inform effective coping strategies.

Seeking professional guidance:

In some cases, assessing stress triggers may require professional guidance. Mental health professionals, such as therapists or counselors, can offer objective insights and support individuals in identifying and addressing their stress triggers. Through therapy, individuals can learn healthy coping mechanisms and develop resilience in the face of stress.

Developing Coping Strategies:

Once stress triggers have been identified, individuals can develop personalized coping strategies to manage stress effectively. These may include practicing relaxation techniques, such as deep breathing or mindfulness meditation, establishing healthy boundaries, seeking social support, or engaging in physical activity. Experimenting with different coping strategies can help individuals determine what works best for them.

Assessing stress triggers is a crucial step in managing stress and promoting emotional well-being. By identifying situational, emotional, and behavioral triggers, individuals can develop personalized coping strategies to mitigate the impact of stress on their lives.

Through self-awareness, reflection, and proactive intervention, individuals can build resilience and lead healthier, more balanced lives.

5.3: Implementing Stress Management Strategies

Implementing stress management strategies involves adopting techniques and habits to reduce stress levels and promote overall well-being. Here are some effective strategies:

1. Mindfulness and Meditation: Practicing mindfulness and meditation can help reduce stress by promoting relaxation and increasing self-awareness. Dedicate a few minutes each day to mindfulness exercises or guided meditation to calm the mind and alleviate stress.

2. Regular Exercise: Engaging in regular physical activity, such as walking, jogging, or yoga, can help reduce stress levels by releasing endorphins and improving mood. Aim for at least 30 minutes

of moderate exercise most days of the week to reap the stress-relieving benefits.

3. Healthy Lifestyle Choices: Prioritize healthy lifestyle habits, including balanced nutrition, adequate sleep, and avoiding excessive caffeine and alcohol consumption. A well-nourished body and sufficient rest can better equip you to handle stressors effectively.

4. Time Management: Develop effective time management skills to prioritize tasks, set realistic goals, and avoid feeling overwhelmed by deadlines and obligations. Break tasks into smaller, manageable steps, and allocate time for relaxation and self-care.

5. Social Support: Maintain strong social connections with friends, family, or support groups. Talking to trusted individuals about your feelings can provide emotional support and perspective, helping to reduce stress levels.

6. Relaxation Techniques: Explore relaxation techniques such as deep breathing exercises, progressive muscle relaxation, or aromatherapy to promote relaxation and reduce muscle tension associated with stress.

7. Setting Boundaries:Learn to set healthy boundaries in your personal and professional lives to prevent burnout and overwhelm. Saying no to tasks or commitments that exceed your capacity can help you manage stress more effectively.

8. Seeking Professional Help: If stress becomes overwhelming or interferes with daily functioning, don't hesitate to seek professional help from a therapist or counselor. They can provide guidance, support, and coping strategies tailored to your individual needs.

9. Engaging in Hobbies:Make time for activities and hobbies that bring you joy and relaxation, whether it's reading, gardening, painting, or playing music. Engaging in enjoyable activities

can distract from stressors and promote a sense of fulfillment.

10. Practice self-compassion:Be kind to yourself and practice self-compassion during times of stress. Recognize that it's okay to feel stressed and that you're doing the best you can. Treat yourself with the same kindness and understanding you would offer to a friend facing similar challenges.

By incorporating these stress management strategies into your daily routine, you can effectively reduce stress levels and cultivate a greater sense of well-being and resilience.

5.4: Timely and Adequate Sex in Optimal Stress Management

Sexual activity can indeed play a role in stress management by promoting relaxation, releasing feel-good hormones like oxytocin and endorphins, and fostering emotional connection with a partner. However, it's essential to emphasize that optimal stress management encompasses a variety of strategies, and sexual activity is just one aspect. Here are some points to consider regarding the role of sex in stress management:

1. Physical Benefits: Engaging in sexual activity can lead to physical benefits such as reduced muscle tension, lower blood pressure, and improved immune function, all of which contribute to overall stress reduction.

2. Emotional Well-Being:Sexual intimacy can enhance emotional well-being by promoting feelings of intimacy, closeness, and connection with a partner. These emotional bonds can provide a sense of support and comfort during times of stress.

3. Stress Relief:Orgasm releases endorphins, which are natural stress relievers, leading to a sense of relaxation and euphoria. This can help alleviate stress symptoms and improve mood.

4. Communication and Bonding:Healthy sexual relationships often involve open communication and mutual trust, which can strengthen the emotional bond between partners. Communicating about sexual needs and desires can foster intimacy and reduce tension in the relationship, contributing to overall stress management.

5. Individual Differences: It's important to recognize that the role of sex in stress management varies from person to person. Some individuals may find sexual activity to be a significant stress reliever, while others may prefer other forms of relaxation or coping mechanisms.

6. Balance and Prioritization: While sex can be a beneficial component of stress management, it's essential to maintain a balanced approach and prioritize other aspects of self-care, such as exercise, relaxation techniques, and social support. Finding a balance that works for you and your partner is key to your overall well-being.

7. Consent and Comfort: It's crucial to engage in sexual activity only when both partners are comfortable and consenting. Pressure or coercion can lead to increased stress and strain on the relationship. Open communication and mutual respect are essential for a healthy sexual relationship.

While sexual activity can be a valuable component of stress management for many individuals, it's essential to approach it as part of a holistic approach to well-being. Communication, consent, and mutual satisfaction are key elements of a healthy sexual relationship that can contribute to overall stress reduction and emotional well-being.

5.5: Monitoring Stress Management Progress

Implementing stress management strategies involves adopting techniques and habits to reduce stress levels and promote overall well-being. Here are some effective strategies:

1. Mindfulness and Meditation:Practicing mindfulness and meditation can help reduce stress by promoting relaxation and increasing self-awareness. Dedicate a few minutes each day to mindfulness exercises or guided meditation to calm the mind and alleviate stress.

2. Regular Exercise:Engaging in regular physical activity, such as walking, jogging, or yoga, can help reduce stress levels by releasing endorphins and improving mood. Aim for at least 30 minutes of moderate exercise most days of the week to reap the stress-relieving benefits.

3. Healthy Lifestyle Choices: Prioritize healthy lifestyle habits, including balanced nutrition, adequate sleep, and avoiding excessive caffeine and alcohol consumption. A well-nourished body and sufficient rest can better equip you to handle stressors effectively.

4. Time Management: Develop effective time management skills to prioritize tasks, set realistic goals, and avoid feeling overwhelmed by

deadlines and obligations. Break tasks into smaller, manageable steps, and allocate time for relaxation and self-care.

5. Social Support: Maintain strong social connections with friends, family, or support groups. Talking to trusted individuals about your feelings can provide emotional support and perspective, helping to reduce stress levels.

6. Relaxation Techniques: Explore relaxation techniques such as deep breathing exercises, progressive muscle relaxation, or aromatherapy to promote relaxation and reduce muscle tension associated with stress.

7. Setting Boundaries: Learn to set healthy boundaries in your personal and professional lives to prevent burnout and overwhelm. Saying no to tasks or commitments that exceed your capacity can help you manage stress more effectively.

8. Seeking Professional Help: If stress becomes overwhelming or interferes with daily functioning, don't hesitate to seek professional help from a therapist or counselor. They can provide guidance, support, and coping strategies tailored to your individual needs.

9. Engaging in Hobbies:Make time for activities and hobbies that bring you joy and relaxation, whether it's reading, gardening, painting, or playing music. Engaging in enjoyable activities can distract from stressors and promote a sense of fulfillment.

10. Practice self-compassion: Be kind to yourself and practice self-compassion during times of stress. Recognize that it's okay to feel stressed and that you're doing the best you can. Treat yourself with the same kindness and understanding you would offer to a friend facing similar challenges.

By incorporating these stress management strategies into your daily routine, you can effectively reduce stress levels and cultivate a greater sense of well-being and resilience.

CHAPTER 6: Effective Stress Management Techniques for Daily Life

In today's fast-paced world, stress has become a common companion in our daily lives. From work pressures to personal challenges, it's crucial to have effective strategies for managing stress. Here are some practical techniques to help you navigate through stress in your daily routine:

1. Mindfulness Meditation: Take a few minutes each day to practice mindfulness meditation. Focus on your breath, observing your thoughts and sensations without judgment. This practice can help calm your mind and reduce stress levels.

2. Physical Activity: Engage in regular physical activity, such as walking, jogging, yoga, or dancing. Exercise releases endorphins, which are natural stress relievers, and helps to clear your mind.

3. Time management: break tasks into smaller, manageable steps and prioritize them based on importance. Set realistic deadlines and avoid overcommitting yourself. Effective time management reduces feelings of being overwhelmed.

4. Healthy Lifestyle Choices: Maintain a balanced diet, stay hydrated, and get enough sleep each night. A well-nourished body is better equipped to handle stress. Limit caffeine and alcohol intake, as they can exacerbate stress levels.

5. Deep Breathing Exercises: Practice deep breathing exercises whenever you feel stressed. Inhale deeply through your nose, hold for a few

seconds, and exhale slowly through your mouth. This technique triggers the body's relaxation response, reducing stress and promoting a sense of calm.

6. Establish boundaries: Learn to say no to tasks or commitments that add unnecessary stress to your life. Set boundaries with work, family, and friends to prioritize your well-being.

7. Seek Support: Don't hesitate to reach out to friends, family, or a professional counselor for support when you're feeling overwhelmed. Talking about your feelings can provide perspective and help alleviate stress.

8. Practice gratitude: Take time each day to reflect on things you're grateful for. Keeping a gratitude journal or simply expressing appreciation for the good things in your life can shift your focus away from stressors.

9. Limit Screen Time: Reduce exposure to digital devices, especially before bedtime. Excessive screen time can contribute to stress and disrupt sleep patterns. Instead, engage in relaxing activities like reading or listening to calming music.

10. Engage in Hobbies: Make time for activities you enjoy, whether it's gardening, painting, playing an instrument, or cooking. Engaging in hobbies provides an outlet for creativity and helps to distract from stressors.

Remember, managing stress is an ongoing process that requires patience and practice. By incorporating these techniques into your daily routine, you can build resilience and better cope with the challenges life throws your way.

6.1: Navigating Stress Management at Work and in Relationships

Stress Management

Managing stress is essential for maintaining overall well-being, especially in two significant areas of life: the workplace and relationships. Here are tailored strategies to effectively handle stress in these domains:

Stress Management at Work:

1. Effective Communication: Clearly communicate with your colleagues and supervisors about workload, deadlines, and expectations. Open communication reduces misunderstandings and prevents stressors from escalating.

2. Break Tasks into Manageable Steps: Break down complex projects into smaller, achievable tasks. This approach prevents feeling overwhelmed and allows for a sense of accomplishment with each completed step.

3. Set Boundaries: Establish boundaries between work and personal life to prevent burnout. Avoid checking emails outside of work hours, and take regular breaks to recharge throughout the day.

4. Time Management: Prioritize tasks based on urgency and importance. Utilize tools like to-do lists or time-blocking techniques to allocate time efficiently. Effective time management minimizes the stress associated with deadlines and multitasking.

5. Seek Support: Don't hesitate to ask for help or clarification when needed. Reach out to coworkers, mentors, or supervisors for guidance and support. Collaborating with others can alleviate stress and foster a sense of teamwork.

6. Practice self-care: Take regular breaks to engage in stress-relieving activities, such as deep breathing exercises, stretching, or short walks. Invest in activities that promote relaxation and rejuvenation during breaks.

7. Mindfulness Practices: Incorporate mindfulness techniques into your workday, such as mindful breathing or short meditation sessions. These practices cultivate awareness and help manage stress reactions effectively.

Stress Management in Relationships:

1. Effective Communication: Practice active listening and express your thoughts and feelings openly with your partner. Clear communication fosters understanding and reduces misunderstandings that can lead to stress in relationships.

2. Set Boundaries: Establish healthy boundaries to maintain individual autonomy and respect within the relationship. Communicate your needs and preferences, and be willing to compromise when necessary.

3. Manage Conflict Constructively: Approach disagreements with a solution-oriented mindset rather than resorting to blame or criticism. Practice empathy and seek to understand your partner's perspective, fostering mutual respect and trust.

4. Quality Time Together: Prioritize quality time with your partner to nurture your bond and create positive experiences. Engage in activities you both enjoy and carve out dedicated time for meaningful connection without distractions.

5. Manage external stressors. Together: Support each other during times of external stress, such as work pressures or family challenges. Work as a team to navigate through difficulties, providing mutual encouragement and reassurance.

6. Maintain individual hobbies and interests.

Encourage each other to pursue individual hobbies and interests that promote personal fulfillment and self-care. Respecting each other's need for time alone fosters independence and strengthens the relationship.

7. Seek professional support if needed. If relationship stress becomes overwhelming or persistent, consider seeking the guidance of a

couples therapist or counselor. Professional support can provide tools and strategies to navigate challenges and strengthen the relationship.

By implementing these strategies, you can effectively manage stress both at work and in your relationships, fostering a healthier and more balanced lifestyle.

6.2: Stress Management Tips for Parents and Students

Parents and students alike often face unique stressors in their respective roles. Here are tailored strategies to help parents and students effectively manage stress:

Stress Management for Parents:

1. Prioritize Self-Care: Take care of your physical and mental well-being by prioritizing self-care activities. Allocate time for exercise, relaxation, and hobbies to recharge and maintain resilience in the face of parenting challenges.

2. Establish Routines: Create structured routines for both yourself and your children to provide a sense of stability and predictability. Consistent schedules for meals, bedtime, and activities can reduce stress for both parents and children.

3. Set realistic expectations: Avoid placing unrealistic expectations on yourself or your children. Recognize that perfection is unattainable, and allow room for mistakes and imperfections in parenting. Celebrate small victories and practice self-compassion.

4. Seek Support: Build a support network of friends, family members, or fellow parents who can offer understanding, advice, and encouragement. Don't hesitate to ask for help when needed, whether it's with childcare, household tasks, or emotional support.

5. Effective Communication: Maintain open and honest communication with your children,

fostering trust and understanding. Encourage them to express their thoughts and feelings, and actively listen without judgment. Effective communication strengthens parent-child relationships and reduces stress.

6. Practice stress-relief techniques: Incorporate stress-relief techniques into your daily routine, such as deep breathing exercises, mindfulness meditation, or yoga. These practices promote relaxation and help you manage stress more effectively.

Stress Management for Students:

1. Time Management Skills: Develop effective time management skills to balance academic responsibilities, extracurricular activities, and personal time. Use tools such as planners or digital calendars to prioritize tasks and allocate time efficiently.

2. Break Tasks into Manageable Steps: Break down large assignments or projects into smaller,

manageable tasks to prevent feeling overwhelmed. Set realistic goals and deadlines for each task, and celebrate progress along the way.

3. Healthy Lifestyle Habits: Maintain a balanced diet, get regular exercise, and prioritize sleep to support overall well-being and academic performance. Avoid excessive caffeine or energy drinks, as they can contribute to stress and disrupt sleep patterns.

4. Utilize Support Resources: Take advantage of support resources available at school, such as tutoring services, counseling centers, or study groups. Don't hesitate to seek help from teachers, academic advisors, or peers when struggling with coursework or personal challenges.

5. Practice self-care: Make time for activities that promote relaxation and stress relief, such as spending time with friends, pursuing hobbies, or engaging in creative outlets. Balancing academic

demands with personal interests is essential for overall well-being.

6. Manage Academic Pressure: Set realistic academic goals and avoid comparing yourself to others. Focus on your own progress and growth, and recognize that setbacks are a natural part of the learning process. Practice self-compassion and seek support from trusted adults or mentors when feeling overwhelmed.

By incorporating these stress management strategies into their daily lives, parents and students can navigate challenges more effectively and maintain a healthier balance between responsibilities and well-being.

CHAPTER 7:Coping With Stressful Situations

Coping with stressful situations can be challenging, but there are strategies to help you navigate through them:

1. Deep Breathing:Take slow, deep breaths to activate your body's relaxation response. Inhale deeply through

your nose, hold for a few seconds, and exhale slowly through your mouth.

2. Mindfulness and Meditation:Practice mindfulness techniques or meditation to help you stay present and calm. Focus on the sensations in your body or observe your thoughts without judgment.

3. Physical Activity: Engage in regular exercise or physical activity to reduce stress and improve your mood. Even a short walk or stretching session can make a difference.

4. Healthy Lifestyle:Maintain a balanced diet, get enough sleep, and limit caffeine and alcohol intake. A healthy lifestyle can help you better cope with stress.

5. Seek Support: Talk to friends, family, or a therapist about what you're going through. Sharing your feelings can provide relief and perspective.

6. Time Management: Break tasks into smaller, manageable steps and prioritize what needs to be done. Organizing your time can reduce feelings of overwhelm.

7. Set Boundaries:Learn to say no to additional commitments or obligations when you're feeling overwhelmed. Setting boundaries is essential for maintaining your well-being.

8. Positive Self-Talk:Challenge negative thoughts and replace them with positive affirmations. Remind yourself of your strengths and past successes.

9. Hobbies and Relaxation:Make time for activities you enjoy, whether it's reading, painting, or listening to music. Engaging in hobbies can provide a much-needed break from stress.

10. Acceptance:Accept that some situations are beyond your control. Focus on what you can change and let go of what you can't.

Remember, coping with stress is a journey, and it's okay to seek help when you need it. Be patient with yourself and prioritize self-care during challenging times.

7.1:Coping with Work And Relationship Stress

1. Set Boundaries: Establish clear boundaries between work and personal life to prevent burnout. Define specific work hours and avoid bringing work-related tasks or concerns home with you. Prioritize self-care activities outside of work to recharge and maintain balance.

2. Prioritize Tasks: Organize your workload by prioritizing tasks based on urgency and importance. Break down larger projects into smaller, manageable tasks and tackle them one step at a time. Effective time management reduces feelings of being overwhelmed and promotes productivity.

3. Communicate Openly: Foster open communication with your supervisor and colleagues about workload, deadlines, and expectations. Express concerns or challenges early on and collaborate on finding solutions together. Effective communication reduces misunderstandings and prevents stressors from escalating.

4. Practice stress-relief techniques: Incorporate stress-relief techniques into your daily routine, such as deep breathing exercises, mindfulness meditation, or short breaks to stretch and relax. Engage in physical activity or hobbies outside of work to release tension and clear your mind.

5. Seek Support: Don't hesitate to reach out to coworkers, mentors, or professional counselors for support when needed. Talking about your feelings and seeking guidance can provide perspective and alleviate stress. Build a support network of trusted individuals who understand the demands of your job.

Managing Relationship Stress:

1. Effective Communication: Maintain open and honest communication with your partner, family members, or friends about your thoughts, feelings, and needs. Practice active listening and empathy, seeking to understand their perspective without judgment. Clear communication fosters trust and strengthens relationships.

2. Set Boundaries: Establish healthy boundaries within your relationships to maintain balance and respect. Communicate your needs and preferences openly, and be willing to negotiate and compromise when necessary. Respecting

each other's boundaries promotes mutual understanding and harmony.

3. Manage Conflict Constructively: Approach disagreements or conflicts with a solution-oriented mindset rather than resorting to blame or criticism. Practice effective conflict resolution techniques, such as active listening, compromise, and finding common ground. Addressing issues openly and constructively strengthens the bond between individuals.

4. Quality Time Together: Prioritize quality time with your partner or loved ones to nurture your connection and create positive experiences. Engage in activities you both enjoy, and carve out dedicated time for meaningful interactions without distractions. Spending quality time together strengthens emotional bonds and reduces stress.

5. Seek professional help if needed. If relationship stress becomes overwhelming or persistent, consider seeking the guidance of a couples

therapist or counselor. Professional support can provide tools and strategies to navigate challenges and strengthen the relationship.

By implementing these strategies, you can effectively manage stress in both your work and relationships, fostering a healthier and more balanced lifestyle. Remember that maintaining open communication, setting boundaries, and prioritizing self-care are key components of managing stress effectively in both domains.

7.2:Strategies for Handling Financial Stress

Financial stress can take a toll on both your mental and physical well-being. Here are practical strategies to help you effectively manage and alleviate financial stress:

Assess Your Financial Situation:

1. Face Your Finances: Start by taking a comprehensive look at your financial situation. Make a list of your income, expenses, debts, and savings. Understanding your financial standing is the first step towards addressing any challenges.

2. Identify stressors: Pinpoint specific financial stressors that are causing you the most anxiety. Whether it's debt, insufficient savings, or unexpected expenses, identifying the root causes of your stress will help you develop targeted solutions.

Create a budget and financial plan.

1. Develop a budget. Create a realistic budget that outlines your monthly income and expenses. Allocate funds for essential expenses such as housing, utilities, groceries, and transportation, while also setting aside money for savings and debt repayment.

2. Cut Unnecessary Expenses: Review your expenses and identify areas where you can cut back. This might include dining out less frequently, canceling unused subscriptions, or finding more affordable alternatives for everyday expenses.

3. Prioritize Debt Repayment: If you have outstanding debts, prioritize repayment by allocating extra funds towards high-interest debt or using debt repayment strategies such as the snowball or avalanche method. Making progress on debt repayment can alleviate a significant source of financial stress.

4. Build an Emergency Fund: Aim to build an emergency fund to cover unexpected expenses or financial emergencies. Start small by setting aside a portion of your income each month until you have built up an adequate buffer.

Manage financial anxiety:

1. Practice mindfulness: Incorporate mindfulness techniques into your daily routine to reduce stress and anxiety related to finances. Focus on the present moment and practice gratitude for what you have rather than dwelling on financial worries.

2. Seek Support: Don't hesitate to seek support from friends, family members, or financial professionals. Talking about your financial concerns with someone you trust can provide emotional support and practical advice.

3. Educate yourself: Take proactive steps to educate yourself about personal finance and money management. There are numerous resources available, including books, online courses, and financial literacy workshops, that can help you improve your financial knowledge and confidence.

Take Action:

1. Set Achievable Goals: Establish realistic financial goals that align with your values and priorities. Whether it's saving for a specific purchase, building a retirement nest egg, or paying off debt, setting clear goals can help you stay focused and motivated.

2. Seek Additional Income: Explore opportunities to increase your income through part-time work, freelance gigs, or passive income streams. Generating additional income can provide a financial cushion and alleviate stress associated with financial instability.

3. Monitor Your Progress: Regularly review your financial progress and make adjustments to your plan as needed. Celebrate small victories along the way and stay committed to your long-term financial goals.

Practice Self-Care:

1. Prioritize Your Well-Being: Remember to prioritize self-care and well-being, even when facing financial challenges. Engage in activities that promote relaxation and stress relief, such as exercise, meditation, or spending time with loved ones.

2. Stay Positive: Maintain a positive mindset and focus on the progress you're making, no matter how small. Cultivate gratitude for what you have and remain optimistic about your ability to overcome financial obstacles.

By implementing these strategies, you can effectively manage and alleviate financial stress, empowering yourself to take control of your financial future and achieve greater peace of mind. Remember that addressing financial stress is a journey, and small steps taken consistently can lead to significant improvements over time.

7.3: Navigating Traumatic Events: Strategies for Coping and Healing

Experiencing a traumatic event can have a profound impact on one's mental, emotional, and physical well-being. Here are effective strategies to help you manage and cope with traumatic events:

Acknowledge Your Feelings:

1. Allow Yourself to Feel: It's important to acknowledge and validate your feelings in response to the traumatic event. Allow yourself to experience a range of emotions, including sadness, anger, fear, or confusion, without judgment.

2. Express Your Emotions: Find healthy ways to express your emotions, whether it's through

talking to a trusted friend or family member, writing in a journal, or engaging in creative outlets such as art or music. Expressing your feelings can help release pent-up emotions and promote healing.

Seek Support:

1. Reach Out for Help: Don't hesitate to reach out for support from friends, family members, or mental health professionals. Talking about your experience with someone you trust can provide validation, comfort, and perspective.

2. Join Support Groups: Consider joining a support group for individuals who have experienced similar traumatic events. Connecting with others who understand what you're going through can provide a sense of belonging and mutual support.

Take care of yourself.

1. Prioritize Self-Care: Make self-care a priority by taking care of your physical, emotional, and spiritual needs. Engage in activities that promote relaxation and well-being, such as exercise, meditation, spending time in nature, or practicing mindfulness.

2. Maintain Healthy Habits: Pay attention to your basic needs, including getting enough sleep, eating nutritious foods, and avoiding excessive alcohol or substance use. Taking care of your physical health can support your resilience and ability to cope with stress.

Practice coping strategies:

1. Use Relaxation Techniques: Incorporate relaxation techniques into your daily routine to reduce stress and promote a sense of calm. Deep breathing exercises, progressive muscle relaxation, or guided imagery can help you relax your body and mind.

2. Grounding Techniques: Practice grounding techniques to stay present and connected to the here and now. Focus on your five senses by noticing things you can see, hear, touch, smell, and taste in your environment.

Seek professional help.

1. Therapy and Counseling: Consider seeking the guidance of a therapist or counselor who specializes in trauma therapy. Therapy can provide you with tools and strategies to process your experience, manage the symptoms of trauma, and work towards healing and recovery.

2. Trauma-Informed Care: Look for mental health professionals who are trained in trauma-informed care and evidence-based treatments for trauma, such as cognitive-behavioral therapy (CBT), eye movement desensitization and reprocessing (EMDR), or trauma-focused cognitive therapy (TF-CBT).

Be patient with yourself.

1. Practice self-compassion: Be gentle and patient with yourself as you navigate the healing process. Healing from a traumatic event takes time, and it's okay to progress at your own pace. Treat yourself with kindness and compassion.

CHAPTER 8:Building Resilience: Strategies for Long-Term Stress Management

In today's fast-paced world, stress has become a constant companion for many. While occasional stress is a natural part of life, long-term exposure to stress can take a toll on both our physical and mental health. Building resilience is key to effectively managing stress over the long term. Here are some strategies to help you maintain long-term stress resilience.

1. Mindfulness and Meditation: Incorporate mindfulness practices and meditation into your daily routine. These techniques can help you stay grounded, manage your emotions, and reduce the negative effects of stress on your body and mind.

2. Healthy Lifestyle Habits: Focus on maintaining a healthy lifestyle by prioritizing regular exercise, nutritious eating, adequate sleep, and avoiding excessive alcohol and caffeine intake. A strong and healthy body can better cope with stressors.

3. Social Support: Cultivate strong social connections with friends, family, and the community. Having a support network can provide emotional reassurance, practical assistance, and a sense of belonging, all of which contribute to resilience in the face of stress.

4. Time Management and Prioritization: Learn to manage your time effectively and prioritize tasks to avoid feeling overwhelmed. Break tasks into

smaller, manageable steps and tackle them one at a time, focusing on progress rather than perfection.

5. Positive Thinking and Gratitude: Foster a positive mindset by practicing gratitude and reframing negative thoughts. Focus on what you're grateful for and try to find silver linings in challenging situations. A positive outlook can help build resilience and buffer against stress.

6. Seeking Professional Help: Don't hesitate to seek professional help if you're struggling to cope with stress. A therapist or counselor can provide valuable tools, strategies, and support tailored to your individual needs.

7. Self-Care Practices: Make self-care a priority by engaging in activities that bring you joy and relaxation. Whether it's reading a book, taking a bath, or spending time in nature, carving out time for self-care can recharge your batteries and build resilience.

8. Flexibility and Adaptability: Cultivate flexibility and adaptability in the face of change and adversity. Life is full of unexpected challenges, but being able to adapt to new circumstances and bounce back from setbacks is essential for long-term stress resilience.

9. Setting Boundaries: Learn to set boundaries and say no to commitments that cause unnecessary stress. Prioritize your own well-being and allocate your time and energy to activities.

8.1: The Path to Wellness: Building Healthy Habits That Stick

Building healthy habits is the cornerstone of a fulfilling and vibrant life. While it may seem daunting at first, incorporating small, sustainable changes into your daily routine can lead to significant improvements in your overall well-being. Here are some effective strategies for building and maintaining healthy habits that stand the test of time:.

1. Start small and be consistent. Rather than trying to overhaul your entire lifestyle overnight, focus on making small, manageable changes one at a time. Choose one habit to work on initially, such as drinking more water or taking a daily walk, and commit to it consistently. Consistency is key to forming new habits.

2. Set Clear and Achievable Goals: Define specific, measurable, and achievable goals for your new habits. Whether it's exercising three times a week, cooking healthy meals at home, or reducing screen time, having clear goals provides direction and motivation.

3. Create a Routine: Incorporate your new habits into your daily routine to make them feel natural and effortless. Whether it's setting a specific time each day for exercise or meal prepping on Sundays, establishing a routine helps reinforce the behavior until it becomes second nature.

4. Track Your Progress: Keep track of your progress to stay motivated and accountable. Whether you use a journal, a habit-tracking app, or a simple calendar, monitoring your consistency and celebrating your achievements along the way can help reinforce the habit.

5. Find Accountability Partners: Share your goals with friends, family, or a supportive community to hold yourself accountable. Having someone to share your successes and challenges with can provide encouragement and motivation to stick with your healthy habits.

6. Focus on Behavior, Not Outcome: Shift your focus from the outcome to the behavior itself. Instead of fixating on losing a certain amount of weight or achieving a specific result, concentrate on the actions that lead to those outcomes, such as eating nutritious meals or exercising regularly.

7. Practice self-compassion: Be kind to yourself and recognize that building healthy habits is a journey with ups and downs. If you slip up or miss a day, don't be too hard on yourself. Instead, acknowledge the setback, learn from it, and recommit to your goals with compassion and determination.

8. Celebrate Milestones: Celebrate your progress and milestones along the way. Whether it's reaching a certain number of consecutive days of exercise or mastering a new healthy recipe, take time to acknowledge and celebrate your achievements as you work towards your larger goals.

9. Stay Flexible and Adapt: Be willing to adapt your approach as needed and stay flexible in the face of challenges or changes in circumstances. Life is unpredictable, and maintaining healthy habits requires adaptability and resilience.

10. Focus on Long-Term Sustainability: Aim for habits that are sustainable in the long run rather

than quick fixes or fad diets. Choose activities and behaviors that you enjoy and that align with your values and priorities, ensuring that your healthy habits become a lasting part of your lifestyle.

Building healthy habits is a journey that requires patience, persistence, and dedication. By starting small, setting clear goals, creating routines, tracking progress, seeking support, and practicing self-compassion, you can establish habits that promote your physical, mental, and emotional well-being for the long term. Remember that every small step counts, and each day is an opportunity to move closer to the vibrant and fulfilling life you deserve.

8.2:Title: Cultivating Resilience: Strategies for Effective Stress Management

Resilience is the ability to bounce back from adversity, adapt to challenges, and thrive in the face of stress. Cultivating resilience is essential for effectively managing stress and maintaining overall well-being. By developing resilience skills, you can navigate life's ups and downs with greater ease and grace. Here are some strategies to help you cultivate resilience in stress management:

1. Develop self-awareness: Start by becoming aware of your thoughts, emotions, and physical sensations in response to stress. Mindfulness practices such as meditation, deep breathing, and body scans can help you tune into your inner experiences and build resilience by enhancing self-awareness.

2. Build a Strong Support Network: Surround yourself with supportive friends, family members, or colleagues who can offer encouragement, guidance, and a listening ear during challenging times. Knowing that you have people you can rely on can bolster your resilience and provide a sense of connection and belonging.

3. Practice Positive Thinking: Cultivate a positive outlook by reframing negative thoughts and focusing on your strengths, accomplishments,

and opportunities for growth. Adopting a growth mindset, which views setbacks as temporary and learning opportunities, can help build resilience in the face of adversity.

4. Maintain Perspective: When faced with stressful situations, step back and gain perspective by considering the bigger picture. Ask yourself whether the situation will matter in the long run and identify aspects that are within your control. Maintaining a sense of perspective can help prevent stress from becoming overwhelming.

5. Foster Flexibility and Adaptability: Embrace change and uncertainty as natural parts of life and cultivate flexibility in your thinking and behavior. Being able to adapt to new circumstances and adjust your approach as needed can enhance resilience and reduce the impact of stressors.

6. Set realistic goals: Break tasks and goals into smaller, manageable steps and set realistic expectations for yourself. Celebrate progress, no

matter how small, and acknowledge your efforts and achievements along the way. Setting achievable goals can boost confidence and resilience.

7. Practice self-care: prioritize self-care activities that nurture your physical, mental, and emotional well-being. Engage in activities you enjoy, such as exercise, hobbies, or spending time in nature, to recharge and replenish your energy reserves. Taking care of yourself is essential for building resilience.

8. Cultivate Problem-Solving Skills: Develop effective problem-solving skills to tackle challenges and find solutions to stressful situations. Break problems down into manageable steps, brainstorm potential solutions, and take decisive action to address issues as they arise. Problem-solving skills are key components of resilience.

9. Learn from Adversity: View setbacks and failures as opportunities for learning and growth. Reflect

on past experiences of overcoming adversity and identify valuable lessons learned. Embracing adversity as a teacher can strengthen resilience and foster a sense of mastery and competence.

10. Seek professional help if needed. If stress becomes overwhelming or persists despite your best efforts, don't hesitate to seek support from a therapist, counselor, or mental health professional. Professional guidance and support can provide additional tools and strategies for managing stress and building resilience.

Cultivating resilience is a lifelong journey that requires practice, patience, and perseverance. By developing self-awareness, building a strong support network, practicing positive thinking, maintaining perspective, fostering flexibility, setting realistic goals, prioritizing self-care, cultivating problem-solving skills, learning from adversity, and seeking professional help if needed, you can strengthen your resilience and navigate life's challenges with greater ease and resilience. Remember that resilience is not about avoiding stress altogether but rather about bouncing back stronger and wiser in the face of adversity.

CHAPTER 9:Taking Control: Strategies for Managing Stress Effectively

Stress is an inevitable part of life, but how we respond to it can make all the difference in our well-being. By taking proactive steps to manage stress, we can regain a sense of control and resilience in the face of life's challenges. Here are some strategies for taking control of your stress:

1. Identify stressors: Start by identifying the sources of stress in your life. These could be work deadlines, relationship conflicts, financial worries, or health concerns. By pinpointing specific stressors, you can develop targeted strategies to address them.

2. Practice mindfulness: Incorporate mindfulness practices into your daily routine to cultivate awareness and presence in the moment. Mindfulness techniques such as meditation, deep

breathing exercises, and body scans can help reduce stress levels and promote relaxation.

3. Set Boundaries: Learn to set boundaries and say no to commitments or activities that cause unnecessary stress. Prioritize your time and energy on tasks that align with your values and goals, and delegate or eliminate tasks that drain you.

4. Time Management: Develop effective time management skills to prioritize tasks and allocate your time efficiently. Break tasks into smaller, manageable steps, set realistic deadlines, and avoid procrastination to reduce feelings of overwhelm and stress.

5. Engage in Physical Activity: Regular exercise is a powerful stress reliever that can help reduce tension, improve mood, and boost energy levels. Find activities you enjoy, whether it's walking, jogging, yoga, or dancing, and make physical activity a regular part of your routine.

6. Practice Relaxation Techniques: Incorporate relaxation techniques into your daily life to counteract the effects of stress on your body and mind. This could include activities such as listening to calming music, taking a warm bath, practicing progressive muscle relaxation, or spending time in nature.

7. Cultivate supportive relationships: Surround yourself with supportive friends, family members, or colleagues who can offer emotional support and practical assistance during times of stress. Sharing your thoughts and feelings with trusted individuals can provide perspective and validation.

8. Limit Screen Time: Set boundaries around your use of technology and social media to prevent information overload and reduce stress levels. Schedule regular breaks from screens, especially before bedtime, to promote relaxation and improve sleep quality.

9. Nourish Your Body: Fuel your body with nutritious foods that support overall health and well-being. Eat a balanced diet rich in fruits, vegetables, whole grains, lean proteins, and healthy fats, and stay hydrated by drinking plenty of water throughout the day.

10. Seek professional help if needed.

If stress becomes overwhelming or persistent, don't hesitate to seek support from a therapist, counselor, or mental health professional. Professional guidance can provide additional tools and strategies for managing stress and improving coping skills.

Taking control of your stress involves a combination of self-awareness, proactive strategies, and support systems. By identifying stressors, practicing mindfulness, setting boundaries, managing time effectively, engaging in physical activity, practicing relaxation techniques, cultivating supportive relationships, limiting screen time, nourishing your body, and seeking professional help if needed, you can empower yourself to manage stress more effectively and lead a healthier, more balanced life. Remember that taking small steps towards stress management can lead to significant improvements in your overall well-being over time.

Conclusion

"Stress Management: The Escape Route From a Silent Killer" offers a comprehensive guide to understanding and navigating the complexities of stress in our modern lives. By shedding light on the detrimental effects of chronic stress and providing practical strategies for managing it effectively, this book empowers readers to take control of their well-being and break free from the grip of the silent killer. From mindfulness practices and time management techniques to setting boundaries and fostering supportive relationships, the tools and insights provided in this book serve as a roadmap to reclaiming peace, balance, and resilience in the face of life's challenges. With the knowledge and strategies outlined in these pages, readers can embark on a journey towards a healthier, happier life, liberated from the pervasive influence of stress.

Stress Management